Fight
Breast Cancer
with Exercise

Dr. Jeff Vallance
Dr. Kerry Courneya

HEALTH & LIFE

Fight Breast Cancer with Exercise

First Printing September 2014
Library and Archives Canada Cataloguing in Publication
Vallance, Jeff, 1977–, author
           Fight breast cancer with exercise / Jeff Vallance and Kerry Courneya.
Includes bibliographical references.
ISBN 978-1-927126-92-9 (pbk.)
           1. Breast—Cancer—Exercise therapy. 2. Breast—Cancer—Physical
therapy. 3. Breast—Cancer—Patients—Rehabilitation. I. Courneya, Kerry
Stephen, 1963–, author II. Title.
RM725.V34 2014   616.99'449062   C2014-903721-X

Project Director: Nancy Foulds
Project Editor: Kathy van Denderen
Cover image: blue leather texture: © Photos.com / Thinkstock
Photo credits: 25: Judy Hobbs: courtesy Judy Hobbs / 42: Dr. John Mackey: Janet Mah, Cross Cancer Institute, Alberta Health Services / 45: Donna Wachowich: courtesy Donna Wachowich / 48: Donna Kohle: courtesy Donna Kohle / 60: Dr. Laura Rogers: Steve Wood, University of Alabama at Birmingham / 70: Dr. Katia Tonkin: Brian Brady, Cross Cancer Institute, Alberta Health Services / 81: Lisa A. Workman: J Shantz Photography / 95: Dr. Jeff Vallance: University of Alberta, Creative Services / 96: Dr. Kerry Courneya: Zoltan Kenwell, Faculty of Physical Education and Recreation, University of Alberta. All other photos courtesy iStock.

Published by
Company's Coming Publishing Limited
87 East Pender Street,
Vancouver, BC, Canada V6A 1S9
Tel: 604-687-5555 Fax: 604-687-5575

www.companyscoming.com

Company's Coming is a registered trademark owned by Company's Coming Publishing Limited

Produced with the assistance of the Government of Alberta, Alberta Multimedia Development Fund.

We acknowledge the financial support of the Government of Canada through the Canada Book Fund (CBF) for our publishing activities.

Canadian   Patrimoine
Heritage   canadien

PC: 27

One of the most exciting developments over the past few years is the proven role of exercise in decreasing fatigue and improving energy for breast cancer patients while on chemotherapy as well as decreasing the risk of recurrent disease for patients diagnosed with early stage breast cancer.

–Dr. Barbara Walley
Southern Alberta Breast Tumor Group Leader
Tom Baker Cancer Centre, Calgary

Disclaimer

Fight Breast Cancer with Exercise is not designed to replace any information or advice received from medical practitioners regarding breast cancer treatment. This book aims to assist your recovery by helping you to look after your overall health and well-being, specifically through physical activity.

If you feel you need further information or advice on medical treatment options, please contact your health care team.

Acknowledgements

Fight Breast Cancer with Exercise was made possible through funding from an Operating Grant from the Canadian Institutes of Health Research.

This resource was supported by an operating grant awarded to Dr. Jeff Vallance from the Canadian Institutes of Health Research. Dr. Vallance is also supported by the Canada Research Chairs program, as well as a Population Health Investigator Award from Alberta Innovates–Health Solutions. He thanks Celeste Lavallee, Registered Dietician, for her input into this resource.

Dr. Kerry Courneya is supported by the Canada Research Chairs Program.

Your Map to Success

Dear Reader

Navigating the different health resources available for breast cancer survivors can be difficult and confusing. Throughout your treatment, you are told what to do, what not to do, what to eat and what support services to take advantage of. Medical research has shown that being active both during and after your treatments is one of the best things you can do for your physical and mental health. So congratulations on taking the first step in learning about the benefits of physical activity!

Physical activity improves the health of women who have been diagnosed with breast cancer. The benefits are seen in women who are receiving chemotherapy and in women who have completed their treatments. And the most recent evidence suggests that physically active survivors live longer and healthier lives with a reduced risk of their cancer returning.

Given the recorded health benefits of physical activity, our goal in writing this book was to develop a resource to help women facing breast cancer treatments as well as those who have completed treatments to be as physically active as possible. And when we say *physically active*, we don't mean training for and running a marathon or doing a triathlon. The scientific evidence consistently shows that physical activity as simple as brisk walking is associated with a variety of positive health outcomes. And that is the focus of this book…walking. Walking is cheap, it's easy to do, it can be done almost anywhere, and most people can do it. If you are new to an active lifestyle, walking is the perfect place to begin.

In our research, we found that tools such as physical activity guides and step pedometers can help breast cancer survivors to start and maintain a healthy level of physical activity. Depending on where you live, it can be difficult to find a fitness centre near you. And it can be a challenge to find the time or money to join a fitness centre. Our hope is that this book will help you enjoy the benefits of physical activity by walking on your own time and on your own schedule.

At times throughout this book we may appear to be overly repetitive when discussing certain points. We do so to ensure that all of our readers will have no trouble understanding our message about the importance of physical activity.

The principles in this book have been scientifically tested in rigorously designed research studies, with results published in several scholarly journals including the *Journal of Clinical Oncology*. We would like to thank the Canadian Institutes of Health Research for their support in allowing us to develop and provide you with this book. And with your participation and feedback, we can continue to make these resources available to other women with breast cancer.

Be proud of yourself. You have truly taken your first step in being proactive about your health!

Dr. Jeff Vallance
Associate Professor and Canada Research Chair
Alberta Innovates–Health Solutions
Population Health Investigator
Faculty of Health Disciplines
Athabasca University

Dr. Kerry Courneya
Professor and Canada Research Chair
Faculty of Physical Education and Recreation
University of Alberta

The Evidence Is Building

Scientific evidence supports the benefits of being physically active during and after breast cancer treatment. Several research studies have examined the impact of physical activity such as cycling, walking, weight lifting and even yoga on the physical, mental and emotional health of women undergoing breast cancer treatment. And yes, each of these activities is beneficial.

We will show you some research data later on that supports the importance of physical activity. Many studies have focused on walking as the main form of physical activity. And the findings are compelling. More specifically, the research has explored the benefits when breast cancer survivors walked in groups. The women in the studies were receiving different types of treatment for their breast cancer. The results of the studies are exciting!

Whether you are currently fighting breast cancer or you have completed your treatments, all breast cancer survivors are encouraged to be physically active.[1,2] More evidence is emerging each day that shows that being physically active during and after your breast cancer treatments is helpful. In fact, an expert roundtable with the American College of Sports Medicine[2] concluded that physical activity is safe during and after cancer treatments and can improve physical functioning, quality of life and cancer-related fatigue.

Even if you weren't an active person before your diagnosis, now is the time to start—it's never too late.

---

1   Doyle, C., et al. (2006). "Nutrition and physical activity during and after cancer treatment. An American Cancer Society guide for informed choices." *CA: A Cancer Journal for Clinicians,* 56, 323–53.

2   Schmitz, K., et al. (2010). "American College of Sport Medicine roundtable on exercise guidelines for cancer survivors." *Med Sci Sports Exerc,* 42, 1409–26.

The scientific evidence shows that physical activity provides the following benefits to survivors.

- ✔ Chemotherapy treatment sessions are better tolerated.
- ✔ Symptoms associated with breast cancer treatment, such as nausea, may be reduced.
- ✔ Quality of life is improved.
- ✔ Daily activities become easier and less tiring.
- ✔ Muscle mass is maintained.
- ✔ Healthy bones and joints are maintained.
- ✔ Fatigue is reduced.
- ✔ The risk of breast cancer returning is reduced.
- ✔ Physical activity contributes to a longer, more fulfilling life.

The benefits listed above are only a few. The next few pages of this guidebook will show you how being active can positively affect both your physical and your mental health—even during your treatment.

Your Mission!

We hope that this book will be a useful resource to help you increase your level of physical activity so that you are physically active for at least 150 minutes per week; in other words, a minimum of 30 minutes a day, five days a week.[3] We hope you will make this goal your mission in achieving the maximum health benefits of physical activity.

In this book, we will refer to three levels of activity (light, moderate and vigorous). We will also suggest ways to achieve the goal of maintaining a *moderate* level of physical activity because studies have shown that this level has the most health benefits.

If you are already meeting the goal of maintaining moderate physical activity, you can increase your level of physical activity in three ways:

1. Increase the *frequency* of your activity (i.e., seven days a week).

2. Increase the *time* spent doing the activity (i.e., 45 minutes per day).

3. Increase the *intensity* at which you are doing the activity (i.e., do more vigorous intensity activities).

It may sound like a lot of physical activity, especially if you are currently going through treatment, but there are a lot of ways you can accumulate that amount.

As mentioned, physical activity can be done at three intensity levels: light, moderate and vigorous.

---

3   Schmitz, K.H., et al. (2010). "American College of Sports Medicine roundtable on exercise guidelines for cancer survivors." *Med Sci Sports Exerc*, 42, 1409–26.

Light Intensity Activities

Going for a slow stroll around the block or carrying out daily household chores are considered light intensity activities. While doing these types of activities, your heart rate stays the same, you do not perspire and it's easy to carry on a conversation if you are walking with a partner.

Moderate Intensity Activities

Moderate intensity physical activity is one level higher than light intensity activity. Moderate intensity activities include a brisk walk (i.e., walking at a pace as though you are late for a doctor's appointment), a hike or walk through the local trails or a friendly game of racquetball.

During these activities, your heart rate is elevated, you begin to perspire and carrying on a conversation with your activity partner is more difficult. The current physical activity guidelines for breast cancer survivors state that survivors should accumulate at least 150 minutes per week of moderate intensity physical activity.[2] The easiest way to achieve your 150 minutes per week is by doing 20 or 30 minutes of moderate intensity activity per day.

Vigorous Intensity Activities

Vigorous intensity activities include swimming laps, running, playing a competitive game of squash or doing cross-country skiing. During these activities, your heart beats rapidly (you can feel your heart pound in your chest), you start to perspire and it is almost impossible to talk because you are out of breath.

If you would rather engage in vigorous types of activities than in moderate activities, the recommendations state you should do these activities for at least 75 minutes each week.[3] If you can, try to build some resistance training (that is, weight lifting) into your activities. As you'll see later in this guidebook, resistance training is beneficial for women undergoing chemotherapy to treat their breast cancer.

You can accumulate your physical activity in a variety of ways. The benefits of physical activity can be gained by doing as little as 10 minutes of activity at a time, at three different times of the day. For example, if you go for a 10-minute walk after breakfast, lunch and supper, you will meet the recommended goal of 30 minutes of physical activity per day. Start at your own pace, and you'll be surprised at how quickly you will progress. Remember, even a small increase in your activity level will be beneficial to your health.

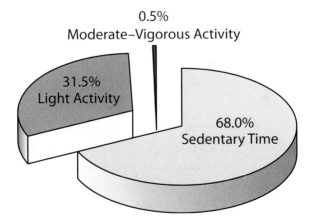

Figure 1: How typical breast cancer survivors spend their day[4]

---

4   Lynch, B.M., Dunstan, D., Vallance, J.K., & Owen, N. (2013). Don't take cancer sitting down: a new survivorship research agenda. *Cancer*, 119, 1928–1935.

By keeping track of your physical activities in a diary or journal, you will be able to see, every day, how much physical activity you are doing, how much progress you have made and how much more you need to do. We have provided a Physical Activity Calendar at the back of this book for your convenience.

Remember to record in your journal the amount of physical activity you do every day—seeing really is believing, and seeing your progress will help motivate you to reach your goals.

It is important to exercise as much as you can to keep muscles working as well as possible. Exercise helps prevent problems that are caused by long-term bed rest, such as stiff joints, weak muscles, breathing problems, constipation, skin sores, poor appetite, and mental changes. It also helps reduce stress and relieve fatigue.

–American Cancer Society

Enhance Your Fitness

One of the many benefits of being physically active is that your fitness level will increase. A breast cancer diagnosis and various treatments (e.g., chemotherapy) are often associated with a drop in fitness. Do you find that climbing a set of stairs is more difficult than when you started treatment? Or that trying to keep up with your kids or grandkids leaves you breathing harder than usual? Your fitness may deteriorate because of the treatments you received, or perhaps you are doing less physical activity than before your diagnosis.

One reason for this decrease in physical activity may have to do with chemotherapy treatment. Some chemotherapy agents can damage your heart and lungs, which can lead to difficulty in carrying out some of your daily tasks or activities. Trying to maintain and increase your fitness both during and after treatment is critical to your well-being and health.

The overwhelming majority of studies indicate that physical activity can help maintain and even improve your fitness both during and after treatment. And you will also feel better. The results are dependent on the types of activities you are doing.

Recently, researchers from across Canada (in Vancouver, Edmonton and Ottawa) conducted the largest study of physical activity in breast cancer survivors specifically receiving chemotherapy.[5] Over 240 newly diagnosed women (who were, on average, 49 years of age) with breast cancer who were receiving chemotherapy participated in this study. The aim of the study was to examine the effects of aerobic training (treadmill or stationary bike) and resistance training (activities such as

---

5   Courneya, K.S., et al. (2007). "Effects of aerobic and resistance exercise in breast cancer patients receiving adjuvant chemotherapy: A multicenter randomized controlled trial." *J Clin Oncol,* 25, 4396–404.

lifting weights) on physical fitness. One group of women (the control group) did not participate in the physical activity intervention. Participants in the exercise intervention groups attended a fitness centre on three days of the week for the duration of their chemotherapy treatments.

The results from this study are compelling! On average, the 78 women who were in the aerobic training group (e.g., walking, jogging, cycling) were able to maintain their cardiovascular fitness throughout their treatments. That is, their heart and lungs were working just as good after their treatments as they were when they started treatment. Stated differently, there was no change in their cardiovascular fitness, whereas the women not doing any physical activity saw a significant decrease in their cardiovascular fitness. This finding is exciting because research shows that chemotherapy is usually associated with reduced cardiovascular fitness.

It's one thing to read about the benefits of physical activity, but it's another thing to see the results! Take a look at Figure 2. If you look at the "aerobic" column (the column on the right), you can see that women participating in the aerobic activity program were able to maintain (and slightly increase) their cardiovascular fitness, while the "inactive" column on the left shows that the women not doing any physical activity saw reduced levels of cardiovascular fitness. The numbers on the left side of the chart (1.0 to –2.5) indicate change in maximal oxygen consumption (the best measure of cardiovascular fitness) as measured in millilitres of oxygen per kilogram of bodyweight per minute (mL/kg/min).

The fact that the women in the aerobic training group even slightly increased their cardiovascular fitness levels is promising given that each woman received a range of four to six months of chemotherapy.

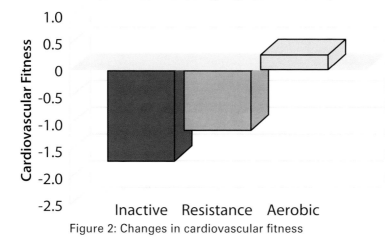

Figure 2: Changes in cardiovascular fitness

In this same study, analysis of the participants' body composition showed that the women who did aerobic activity were able to prevent weight gain while resistance trainers increased their muscle mass. On average, the 82 women in the resistance training group were able to increase their muscular strength (both upper and lower body) by 25 to 30 percent from their pre-study strength.

This result is certainly important given the negative effect of obesity on cancer survival and recurrence. That is, being overweight or obese is linked to a higher likelihood of having a cancer recurrence.[6] The scientific research consistently shows that being healthy (being physically active and eating healthy) and controlling your weight can help you live longer and even reduce the risk of the cancer coming back.

Figure 3 shows that the women participating in the resistance training program actually added over 1 kilogram (2.2 pounds)

---

6   Demark-Wahnefried, W., et al. (2012). "The role of obesity in cancer survival and recurrence." *Cancer Epidemiol Biomarkers Prev, 21*, 1244–59.

of muscle. In addition, even the women doing aerobic training showed an increase in muscle mass. And not surprisingly, the women who did not participate in either of the programs did not show any change in muscle mass.

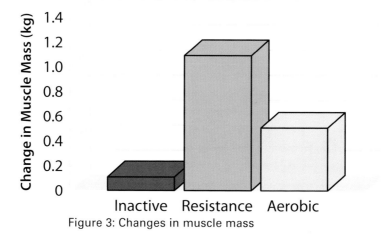

Figure 3: Changes in muscle mass

The scientific research consistently shows that being healthy (being physically active and eating healthy) and controlling your weight can help you live longer and even reduce the risk of the cancer coming back.

But What About Lymphedema?

If you have undergone breast cancer surgery, or even if you are well past your treatments, you may feel like you have limited use of your arm. You may also have some swelling in your arm as a result of lymphedema. Lymphedema is a common side effect of breast surgery when some of the lymph nodes are removed, and it is characterized by a painful swelling and fluid build-up in the arm. This side effect often makes women feel as though they should limit the use of the affected arm.

Until recently, women have been advised not to perform any weight-lifting activities (for example, lifting small children or heavy bags) for fear that it may worsen lymphedema. It was commonly believed that lifting heavy objects and increasing the movement of the affected arm would make the condition worse.

Several research studies recently published on the impact of weight lifting on lymphedema show that physical activity, including weight lifting, is not harmful.[7, 8, 9] In other words, physical activity does not increase the chances of developing lymphedema and does not make the condition worse. These studies have found that weight lifting (at the gym, for example) is safe—it won't cause lymphedema, and it won't make it worse if you already experience lymphedema in one or both arms.

7   Ahmed, R.L., et al. (2006). "Randomized controlled trial of weight training and lymphedema in breast cancer survivors." *J Clin Oncol,* 24, 2765–72.

8   Schmitz, K.H., et al. (2010). "Weight lifting for women at risk for breast cancer–related lymphedema: A randomized trial." *JAMA,* 304, 2699–705.

9   Courneya, K.S., et al. (2007).

If you decide to lift weights as part of your physical activity program, be sure to start with small weights and a low number of repetitions (few lifts). Then gradually build up the weight and repetitions. It may be helpful to learn proper weight-lifting techniques from a qualified trainer. But you don't need expensive weight-lifting machines—items around your home, such as large soup cans, can be just as effective. If you do have symptoms of lymphedema, see a physiotherapist. He or she may recommend that you wear a compression garment on your arm during weight lifting.

Overall, from what we know so far from the research on weight lifting and lymphedema, there is no reason breast cancer survivors can't engage in weight lifting as part of their physical activity routine.

Research Snapshot: Weight Lifting and Lymphedema

A study[10] recently published in the *New England Journal of Medicine* followed breast cancer survivors who had lymphedema. The participants were involved in a one-year weight training program. Women in this study were compared to a group of breast cancer survivors who did not participate in the weight training program. This study found that weight-lifting participants increased their upper and lower body strength. And most importantly, there was no difference in limb and hand swelling between the two groups.

You might ask yourself, "But what about lifting weights while I am on chemotherapy?" Our research team recently published data from an experimental study answering that very question. This 2007 study (mentioned earlier)[11] involved newly diagnosed women with breast cancer who were receiving chemotherapy. There were 82 women who participated in a weight lifting program three days a week for the duration of their chemotherapy, which ranged from four to six months. The results concluded that weight lifting (or other types of physical activity, for that matter) did not cause lymphedema, nor did weight lifting make lymphedema worse.

This study added to the body of research evidence that suggests that weight training (or lifting heavy objects) does not exacerbate lymphedema symptoms. Overall, from what we know so far from the research on weight lifting and lymphedema, there is no reason breast cancer survivors can't engage in weight lifting as part of their physical activity routine.

---

10   Schmitz, K., et al. (2009). "Weight lifting in women with breast cancer–related lymphedema." *NEJM*, 361, 664–73.

11   Courneya, K.S., et al. (2007).

Physical Activity and Chemotherapy Treatments

The same study in 2007[12] found that women who were physically active were able to complete more of the chemotherapy treatments that their oncologist prescribed for them. Oncologists try to deliver at least 85 percent of the chemotherapy that is prescribed for a patient.[13, 14] The research shows that there is a link between a survivor who has achieved her higher dose of chemotherapy prescription and a reduced chance of the breast cancer coming back, as well as improved survival. And these data suggest that being physically active might help survivors tolerate their chemotherapy and achieve the prescription of the oncologist.

In particular, women receiving chemotherapy who were in the weight-training activity group received on average 90 percent of their chemotherapy prescription whereas the group of women not participating in any type of physical activity completed on average 84 percent of their prescription. Women in the aerobic activity group received on average 87 percent of their chemotherapy prescription. The six percent difference between the inactive group and the weight-training activity group was statistically significant; it was not just by chance that this difference was observed.

---

12   Courneya, K.S., et al. (2007).

13   Budman, D.R., et al. (1998). "Dose and dose intensity as determinants of outcome in the adjuvant treatment of breast cancer: The cancer and leukemia group B." *J Natl Cancer Inst,* 90, 1205–11.

14   Wood, W.C., et al. (1994). "Dose and dose intensity of adjuvant chemotherapy for stage II, node-positive breast carcinoma." *NEJM,* 330, 1253–59.

We can present the numbers in a different way. Figure 4 shows the percentage of women in each study group that achieved at least 85 percent of their chemotherapy treatments.

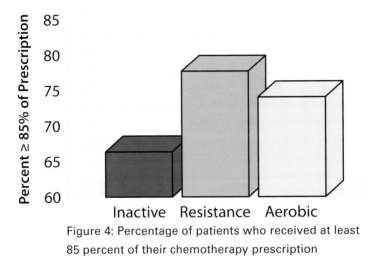

Figure 4: Percentage of patients who received at least 85 percent of their chemotherapy prescription

...being physically active might help survivors tolerate their chemotherapy and achieve the prescription of the oncologist.

Judy Hobbs, 57 (January 2013)

I discovered a lump in my breast in June 2012. I was diagnosed with invasive ductal adenocarcinoma, stage II, grade 3. I had a lumpectomy and sentinel node dissection in early August, followed by four chemotherapy treatments, and I have completed 18 of 25 radiation treatments.

I'm not athletic, but I have always been active. Prior to my diagnosis, I participated in jazzercise classes two or three times a week, and I had an annual membership at a fitness facility that I used sporadically for doing aerobic exercise and weight training. As well, my husband and I went for regular one-hour brisk walks Sunday mornings. I started tennis lessons twice a week in May 2012 and continued with a few more lessons following my lumpectomy.

I knew I was going to lose my hair after my first chemotherapy treatment, so I was apprehensive about working out at a public fitness centre. But I quickly learned about the numerous free fitness programs available for cancer patients in Calgary. I began participating in circuit classes, stretching and aerobic activity with the Beauty Program at the Thrive Centre at the University of Calgary when I started my cancer treatment. I'm comfortable working out with other women with breast cancer; it's very motivating, and I feel energized following my workouts.

My husband and I continued to go for walks, which we modified on days that I felt tired, weak or if I had any pain in my feet and legs. I didn't experience any nausea during my chemotherapy treatments, and other side effects were minimal. I truly believe this is partly due to the physical activity I did every week.

In February 2013 I begin dry-land training once a week with the Sistership Dragon Boat team for breast cancer survivors. In May, when the ice has melted on the Glenmore Reservoir, I will be training on the water twice a week with the team. I'm excited to try a sport I've never done before and be part of a team for the first time in my life! I know I will improve my core and upper body strength, and I look forward to making new friends.

I think the key to being active during cancer treatment is to find an activity that you enjoy, that is affordable and fits into your lifestyle during and after treatment.

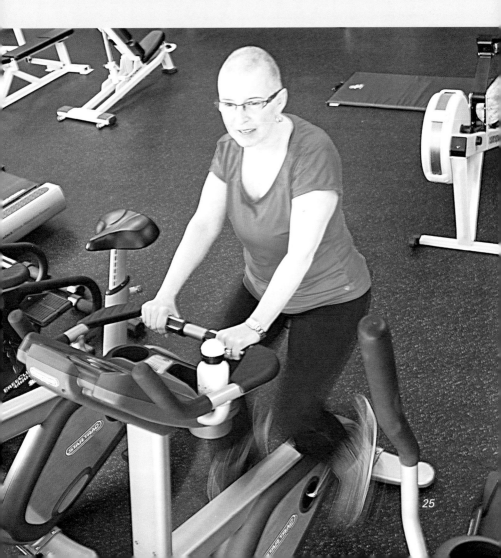

The Benefits of Physical Activity

Keeping Your Mind Off Cancer

Do you ever find yourself worrying about your cancer? Do you ever worry that your cancer will come back? Sometimes breast cancer patients have these and other recurring thoughts related to their diagnosis. Physical activity is a great way to distract yourself from the day-to-day worries about your cancer coming back and any lingering side effects you might experience. Women going through treatments, as well as survivors who have finished their treatments, have told us many times that physical activity helps them to get their mind off their cancer. Even if you are active for just a few minutes, that brief reprieve might be all you need.

When you are physically active, listen to your breathing and try to hear your heart beat. Doing this will help you focus on what you are doing and keep other thoughts at bay. It also helps to do a physical activity in a setting that stimulates you. For example, you may feel more motivated to walk outside enjoying nature than using a treadmill inside your home or gym.

The environment in which you are physically active can make the difference between whether you stop being active or you persist and continue to be active. Find a physical activity you can do in an area and space that makes you want to come back for more. Taking a walk in a local park or shopping mall with a coffee shop nearby is an excellent way to keep motivated—you can stop for a beverage after your stroll!

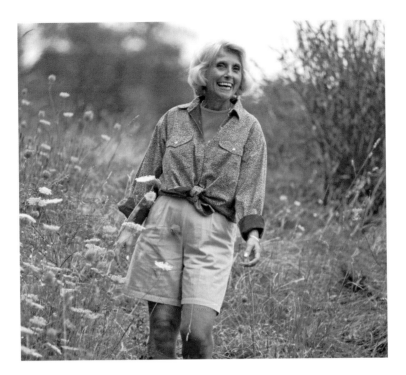

Some running stores provide maps of local walking trails around your neighbourhood. They may also have walking programs that will help you to find partners or groups to walk with. Browse the newsletters or bulletins in your community to see what physical activity programs are offered.

Physical activity is a great way to relieve stress. When you are physically active, you are doing something that distracts you from any challenges you may face during the day, even if the stressors are not related to your diagnosis and treatments. Physical activity can relax tense muscles and help you sleep better. Physical activity can also decrease stress hormones, such as cortisol, and increase endorphins. Endorphins are your body's "feel good" chemicals that boost your mood naturally (much like the "runner's high").

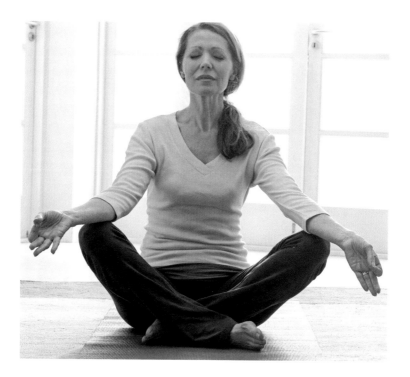

Keep in mind that any type of physical activity is beneficial. You don't have to walk, jog or cycle. Interested in yoga? Some yoga programs are targeted toward cancer survivors. Exciting research from the Faculty of Kinesiology at the University of Calgary has explored the effects of yoga on women with breast cancer.[15] This research has found that survivors participating in a seven-week yoga program reported fewer symptoms of stress at the end of the program.

These same researchers recently published a comprehensive review on yoga for cancer survivors and concluded that clinically significant changes in various health outcomes indicate that yoga is a promising activity for improving cancer survivors'

15 Culos-Reed, S.N., et al. (2006). "A pilot study of yoga for breast cancer survivors: Physical and psychological benefits." *Psycho-Oncology,* 15, 891–97.

health and well-being.[16] Too often we might think physical activity is limited to jogging on a treadmill or going to the local gym to workout. But really, the types of physical activities available to you are endless—go out and explore…or strike a pose!

Your Energy Level Is Improved

One of the most studied health factors in the field of physical activity and cancer is fatigue. Fatigue is the most common and distressing side effect reported by women receiving treatment for breast cancer. The National Cancer Institute (www.cancer.gov) reports that at least 70 percent of patients list fatigue as the symptom most associated with their cancer treatments.

Breast cancer treatments can cause women to feel tired and have a lack of energy. And these feelings of fatigue can last well after their last treatment. Making the problem worse is that fatigue tends to increase as sedentary activities become more common. Sedentary activities include a lot time spent sitting, such as watching television or using a computer. This lack of energy may limit your ability to do the daily activities that you once found easy to carry out.

Several studies have shown that breast cancer survivors who are physically active have decreased symptoms of tiredness, and they have more energy.[17] One recently published overview of all the physical activity and cancer-related fatigue studies concluded that aerobic exercise (such as brisk walking, jogging and cross-country skiing) is beneficial for people with, and who have had cancer.[16] The researchers identified a total of 56 studies that have

---

16 Culos-Reed, S.N., et al. (2012). "Yoga and cancer interventions: A review of the clinical significance of patient reported outcomes for cancer survivors." *Evid Based Complement Alternat Med,* Epub ahead of print.

17 Cramp, F., and Dyron-Daniel, J. (2012). "Exercise for the management of cancer-related fatigue in adults." *Cochrane Database Syst Rev,* Nov 14, CD006145.

examined the impact of physical activity on fatigue levels. And we also know that the more sedentary a survivor is, the more symptoms of fatigue she will experience.

Physical activity helps reduce feelings of tiredness in many ways. It helps your red blood cells work better. Red blood cells carry oxygen throughout your body, and when you are not active, your body does not use oxygen efficiently. When you are physically active, you increase the ability of your body to use oxygen in the blood, and you feel more energized as a result.

What About Depression?

Many breast cancer survivors experience symptoms of depression during treatments and even after treatments have finished. There are several ways you can prevent depression from creeping up on you or help manage depression if you are experiencing symptoms. For example, some therapies that have been shown to be helpful for depression among cancer survivors include group psychotherapy, educational resources, art therapy, music therapy and individual one-on-one counselling.

While these programs do have some small positive effects on depression (and other psychosocial health outcomes), they are unlikely to also address the physical and functional concerns experienced by many breast cancer survivors. Many survivors report feeling fatigue, for example, or they may have other physical or functional limitations. Physical activity can help alleviate both the emotional and the physical symptoms of depression.

One thing that has been found to enhance both the physical and psychosocial health of cancer survivors is, indeed, physical activity. Clinically relevant and exciting evidence continues to emerge that supports the role of physical activity as a safe and effective intervention to prevent depression and reduce depression symptoms.[18, 19]

If you are feeling a little bit down and blue, some physical activity can lift your spirits. The scientific data supports this fact. One recent research study examined over 40 different physical activity interventions and found that being active was related to reduced symptoms of depression.[18] In other words, physically active patients reported having fewer depressive symptoms.

During one study involving 483 rural breast cancer survivors who were post-treatment, Dr. Laura Rogers and her colleagues found that those survivors who reported no leisure-time physical activity had significantly higher depression scores compared to those survivors who were accruing at least 150 minutes per week of at least moderate intensity physical activity.[19]

This study also explored whether there was any relationship between the amount of time survivors spent sitting and depression. The direction of the data supported a positive trend between sitting time and depression symptoms. We should note, however, that there are several ongoing studies examining the relationship between sedentary behaviour and depression among cancer survivors.

You May Live Longer

You're never too old to increase your level of physical activity. It has been found that if you are physically active, your body actually tends to age slower. And some exciting research with

18   Brown, J.C., et al. (2012). "The efficacy of exercise in reducing depressive symptoms among cancer survivors: A meta-analysis." *PLoS One,* 7, Epub.

19   Rogers, L.Q., et al. (2011). "Physical activity type and intensity among rural breast cancer survivors: Patterns and associations with fatigue and depressive symptoms." *Journal of Cancer Survivorship*, 5(1), 54–61.

breast cancer survivors is now suggesting that physically active survivors live longer.[20, 21, 22, 23] One study in the *Journal of the American Medical Association* showed that breast cancer survivors who walked briskly for three to five hours per week significantly reduced their chances of dying from breast cancer compared to survivors who were not active.[20]

Figure 5 shows that the survivors who walked at a moderate intensity for three to five hours per week had the highest risk reduction of death—the risk reduction was approximately 50 percent.[20] As you can see, you don't have to do an excessive or unreasonable amount of walking to reap these benefits. It's as simple as taking a brisk walk for 30 to 45 minutes each day.

Furthermore, this study found that being active at higher intensities was not significant. In other words, the greatest benefit came from moderate intensity activities done for three to five hours per week (see Figure 5). So, as indicated earlier, anyone can maintain a good level of physical activity—you don't need to run a marathon to be physically fit.

Of course, this does not mean you should avoid more vigorous activities. Vigorous activities were still beneficial in helping survivors live longer because any level of physical activity has benefits.

As another example, Dr. Christine Friedenreich and her team[21] in Alberta followed over 1200 breast cancer survivors and found that moderate intensity physical activity (walking

20 Holmes, M., et al. (2005). "Physical activity and survival after breast cancer diagnosis." *JAMA*, 293, 2479–86.

21 Friedenreich, C.M., et al. (2009). "Prospective cohort study of lifetime physical activity and breast cancer survival." *Int J Cancer*, 124, 1954–62.

22 Irwin, M., et al. (2008). "Influence of pre- and postdiagnosis physical activity on mortality in breast cancer survivors: The health, eating, activity, and lifestyle study." *J Clin Onc*, 20, 3958–64.

23 Holick, C., et al. (2008). "Physical activity and survival after diagnosis of invasive breast cancer." *Cancer Epidemiol Biomarkers Prev*, 17, 379–86.

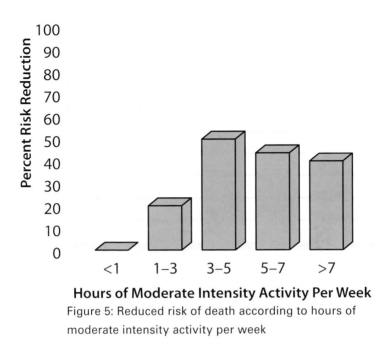

Figure 5: Reduced risk of death according to hours of moderate intensity activity per week

like you were late for an appointment) reduced the risk of a breast cancer recurrence and increased survival. This study showed that all levels of physical activity are valuable.

Dr. Friedenreich's study found that even the physical activity you did in the years before your diagnosis is helpful. That is, survivors who were physically active on a regular basis even before they were diagnosed with breast cancer had a reduced risk of recurrence and survival. However, it is important to repeat here that even if you have been inactive, it is never too late to start to increase your physical activity.

Researchers at Yale University found that the physical activity you do *after* your treatment may be more important than the activity you do *during* your treatment.[22] Among a group of 933 breast cancer survivors who completed treatment, it was found that the women who increased their physical activity

...survivors who walked at a moderate intensity for three to five hours per week had the highest risk reduction of death... approximately 50 percent....It's as simple as taking a brisk walk for 30 to 45 minutes each day.

after diagnosis had a 45 percent lower risk of death, whereas survivors who decreased their physical activity after diagnosis had a four-fold greater risk of death.

The results of these studies are powerful. They are the first studies to show that physical activity has a relevant and clinical impact on the long-term health and survival of women diagnosed with breast cancer. From what the science of medicine knows so far, being physically active is one of the most effective ways to reduce your risk of your breast cancer coming back, and it can increase your chances of a longer and healthier life free of cancer.

Many doctors now encourage people with cancer to be as active as possible during treatment and recovery.

–Canadian Cancer Society

The Risk of Cancer Recurrence Is Reduced

We know that regular physical activity may lower the risk of getting breast cancer. And we know that active survivors have a higher chance of living longer than inactive survivors. Not only do active survivors live longer, but they also have a lower chance of their cancer coming back.[20]

The *Journal of the American Medical Association* study (mentioned earlier) also found that survivors who were active between three and five hours per week at a moderate intensity had a 43 percent reduced risk of their breast cancer returning later in life.[20] And remember, moderate intensity activity is the equivalent of brisk walking (like you were late for an appointment). All levels of activities (light, moderate, vigorous) are helpful, but the research shows that the advantages (decreased recurrence and increased survival) can be achieved by simply getting out for a walk on at least three days of the week.

What is it about physical activity that helps women live longer and reduces the chances of their breast cancer recurring? One reason is that physical activity has been shown to positively influence estrogen levels and insulin resistance in survivors (insulin monitoring is important even if you are not diabetic), which may prevent a cancer recurrence.

A great deal of research has explored the role of weight and weight gain after a diagnosis of breast cancer. One study has shed light on this relationship.[24] A team of researchers studied 5000 breast cancer survivors and found that women can help protect themselves against their cancer returning by maintaining a healthy body weight. And we know that regular physical activity can help survivors achieve and maintain a healthy body weight.

---

24 Kroenke, C., et al. (2005). "Weight, weight gain, and survival after breast cancer diagnosis." *J Clin Onc*, 23, 1370–78.

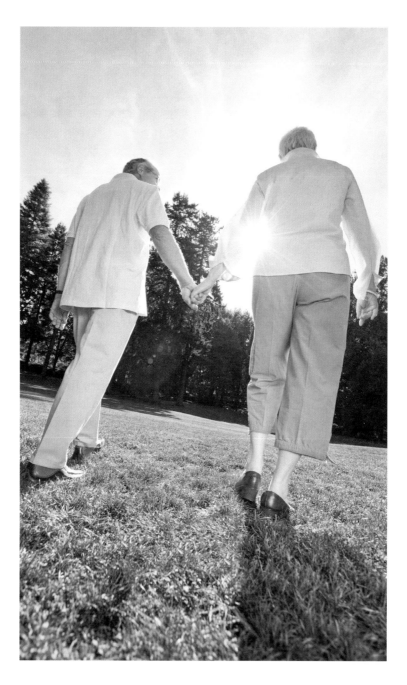

Getting Support for Activity

You might find it difficult to start or maintain a physical activity program on your own. Sometimes we all need some encouragement or a helping hand to get us started or keep us motivated to continue.

One of the reasons most people are not physically active is that it is often difficult to dedicate yourself to a program of physical activity. Finding the time to devote to physical activity might be problematic for reasons unrelated to cancer. There are so many things that prevent us from being active. You might be involved with your kids' after-school activities, your job may be busy, or the weather might prevent you from being active. Or let's face it, you just might not be motivated to be physically active.

However, the research tells us that having a trusted social support network is one of the strongest influences on whether people are active or not. As you read on, think of the people within your social circle, such as your friends or family members, that can join you during your physical activity. The power of two is always stronger than the power of one! And having a partner to share and talk with during your physical activity is enjoyable and will help keep you motivated. You may even find that you look forward to your next walk!

Two Is Better Than One!

If you are one of those people that like to plug in your iPod and do a physical activity on your own, that's great! But sometimes we can't go it alone. Many survivors find it more enjoyable to do an activity with a partner. Your spouse, partner or a friend can help motivate you to be active.

Can you think of certain individuals in your life that can help you be active? Invite a support person to be physically active with you. Then you can both enjoy the benefits of physical activity. Complete the goal-setting activity on pages 64 to 67, which will help get you started. Set at least one goal together.

Encourage each other to set physical activity targets, and hold each other accountable for meeting these goals. Remember to celebrate when you achieve your goals.

ACTIVITY 1

Name three people that you think can help motivate you to get active:

1. _____

2. _____

3. _____

ACTIVITY 2

List some of the activities that you and your support person/people enjoy doing together:

1. _____

2. _____

3. _____

Family Matters

Getting the support of your family to be physically active is a good way to start and help you maintain your program. Here are some tips to help get your family active.

- ✔ Take lessons together in a new sport, such as tennis or golf.
- ✔ Take a walk or go for a bike ride in your neighbourhood.
- ✔ Go to the nearest park and play games, such as softball, soccer or volleyball.
- ✔ Go for a hike in a nature preserve or park. Bring a book about local wildlife or flowers with you so you and your family can identify birds and plants on your hike.
- ✔ Jump rope. It's a great physical activity and it can be done almost anywhere.

All types of physical activity count!

An active family is a happy family! You can even include physical activity in the daily routine you and your family engage in. Have you and your spouse ever thought about riding your bikes to work instead of taking the car? Or walking to the grocery store?

Physical activity can be a great way to bond with your family. Now is your chance to be an example to your family and help them to be physically active as well. Encourage your clan to go for a walk after dinner. Alternatively, depending on the season, you can take your children or grandchildren bike riding or skating at a local ice rink. Most kids won't turn down those opportunities!

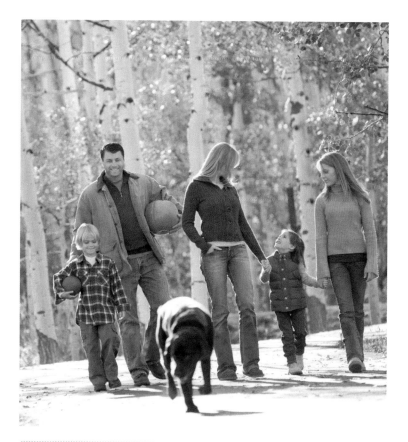

ACTIVITY 3

Think of three activities that you can do with your family over the next month, regardless of the season:

1. _____

2. _____

3. _____

ACTIVITY 4: FAMILY ACTIVITY TIME

Write down one time each day when you can be active with your family:

Monday: _____

Tuesday: _____

Wednesday: _____

Thursday: _____

Friday: _____

Saturday: _____

Sunday: _____

Now write down the activities your family can all do together on these days:

Monday: _____

Tuesday: _____

Wednesday: _____

Thursday: _____

Friday: _____

Saturday: _____

Sunday: _____

Dr. John Mackey

The studies that are emerging in the physical activity and cancer area are very supportive of the role that physical activity can play both during and after your breast cancer treatments. Here in our clinic, we place a lot of emphasis on continuing to be active both during and after breast cancer treatments. We have found that an active lifestyle can improve your physical fitness and your quality of life.

There is very exciting and clinically relevant data being published indicating that breast cancer survivors who are physically active have a reduced risk of having their cancer return. And we are finding that active survivors live longer and healthier lives compared to survivors who are not active. These studies show that you don't need to be training for marathons to get these benefits. It's as simple as getting out for walk.

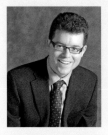 I, and many of my colleagues, recommend patients regularly engage in physical activity. And I recommend my patients do their best to stay active as much as possible even while they are going through treatments. We have data showing that all types of physical activities are helpful. If you are not sure where to start, I encourage you to drop in to your local fitness centre, or ask your oncologist or a member of your health care team, such as a physiotherapist. It's never too late to start being active. You'll notice the benefits immediately.

–Dr. John Mackey is a medical oncologist and the director of the Breast Cancer Program at the Cross Cancer Institute in Edmonton, Alberta. Dr. Mackey is also the executive director of the Cancer International Research Group

You've Got a Friend

Friends can be the biggest motivator to be healthy. When it comes to physical activity, research indicates that people who are active with friends are much more likely to stick to their activity routine compared to people who are active alone.

If some of your friends are not physically active, share this guide with them. If you have friends that already are active, ask to join them. Friends can be a great source of advice. Try to surround yourself with role models and supportive people who will help and encourage you to be active. If you interact with people who are healthy and active, odds are it will be easier for you to stay active as well. Peer pressure is a wonderful thing if you use it in positive ways!

Have fun with your friends by forming a walking group. Meet once or twice a week at a convenient location and walk around your favourite park. Gather your friends and join in a Learn-to-Run class. Many running and walking stores offer clinics on walking, jogging and marathons and have several programs to suit what you are looking for and that match your activity level.

If some of your friends are not physically active, share this guide with them.... Peer pressure is a wonderful thing if you use it in positive ways!

Donna Wachowich (January 2013)

I was diagnosed with breast cancer in January 2011 at the age of 52. The tumour was small but rapidly growing (grade 3), so I was treated with lumpectomy, chemotherapy and radiation.

I took on a physical activity program (the Beauty Program) at the Thrive Centre at the University of Calgary in July 2011 during my course of treatment between radiation and chemotherapy. It helped to reduce the post-treatment fatigue and kept me feeling positive and motivated in that I was doing something in addition to the medical treatment to reduce the risk of cancer recurrence.

I have stayed active by continuing in the Beauty Program at the Thrive Centre, and I also joined the Sistership Dragon Boat team in 2012. I have also continued doing other activities I enjoy, including curling, cycling, walking and hiking in the mountains.

My main barrier to keeping active is a very busy life and career as a family doctor. I took a medical leave from early 2011 to early 2012 and returned to work on a part-time basis. However, it still seems to be a challenge to fit exercise into my schedule!

The advice I would give to others is to put regular exercise commitments into your schedule as if they are appointments. Consider exercise to be part of your ongoing cancer treatment, and connect with at least one exercise buddy to keep each other motivated to maintain your commitment to regular physical activity.

"...connect with at least one exercise buddy to keep each other motivated to maintain your commitment to regular physical activity.

Your Physical Activity Prescription

The Recommended Goal

The goal for you is to increase your level of physical activity so that by the end of your chemotherapy, you achieve a moderate level of activity on at least five days of the week, for a minimum of 30 minutes each day (for 150 minutes each week). Or if vigorous activity is your choice, do this on three days of the week for a minimum of 20 minutes each time.

Remember, start slowly and work your way up to the recommended amount of physical activity.

If you are already meeting this moderate level of physical activity goal, you can try to increase the frequency of your activity (i.e., seven days a week), increase the time spent doing the activity (i.e., increase to 45 minutes) and increase the intensity at which you are doing the activity (i.e., do more vigorous intensity activities).

How Often Should I Be Physically Active?

If you choose a moderate intensity physical activity (like brisk walking), being active on at least five days of the week is optimal for health benefits. This might seem hard to achieve, but we will give you some helpful tips on how to reach that goal. If you are doing (or would rather do) vigorous intensity physical activities instead of moderate activity, you should try to do these activities on three days of the week.

How Much Do I Have to Sweat?

So now the bad news: you have to sweat a little bit. It is important to get your heart rate up and your lungs and heart working! But you don't have to exhaust yourself. If you want to sustain your physical activity routine, it needs to be enjoyable. Try to be physically active at least at a moderate intensity.

Moderate intensity physical activity is any activity that makes you breathe harder without feeling out of breath. If you are active at a moderate intensity, you should start to sweat after 10 minutes. If someone were to see you walking at a moderate intensity, they would think you were late for an appointment. Have you ever wanted to escape from a busy crowd at the shopping mall? Now that's a good example of brisk walking!

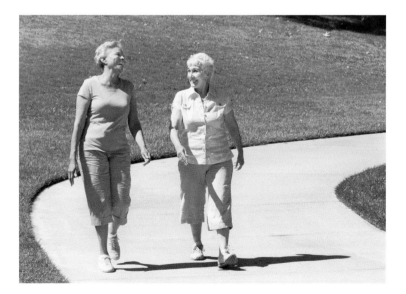

Donna Kohle (January 2013)

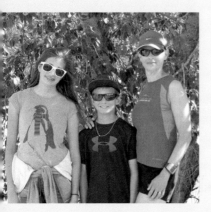

Prior to my diagnosis of breast cancer I was a healthy and active mother of an 11- and 14-year-old. I enjoyed a variety of physical activities but used running as my main form of exercise.

Soon after my diagnosis, I started treatment, which included a partial mastectomy and sentinel node biopsy. This surgery showed that the cancer had spread to my lymph nodes. I underwent chemotherapy and radiation as well as starting on a five-year protocol of the drug Tamoxifen. Unfortunately, I developed lymphedema in my left arm as a result of my treatment.

Because physical activity was already an important part of my life, I had hoped to continue to be active while undergoing treatment. But I was unsure of what types of physical activity would be appropriate and was worried that I may not feel well enough to exercise. My oncologist encouraged me to stay active. She assured me that this would help alleviate some of the side effects of treatment.

My exercise routine took on a new gentler approach in the form of walking and yoga. On the days when I was feeling the worst—weak, nauseated and in pain—that would mean just shuffling around my house or backyard. On days when I would be feeling slightly better, with more energy, I would take my dog for long walks in nearby Nosehill Park, often accompanied by a friend or family member. I can honestly say that I always felt better once I started moving regardless of how small the movement was. It was a great distraction from the pain and nausea. It also gave me a sense of accomplishment.

I was lucky enough to find an exercise program specifically designed for cancer patients and have continued through my recovery with this program. I found it comforting to be surrounded by people going through the same challenges as I was. Also, it gave me confidence in my ability to help fight the disease.

It was often difficult to get up from the couch and get moving when I wasn't feeling well, but it was exactly what I needed to do to help myself. During treatment, we are constantly being told what we have to do—blood tests, scans, surgery, chemotherapy, radiation, drugs. Exercise is a way to take back some control over our bodies and the cancer we are fighting.

Besides giving me more control over this awful disease, physical activity helped lessen the severity of the side effects of treatment. I had more energy, and just as important for both my family and myself, it kept me more mentally balanced!

As I moved into the recovery phase, I continued to stay active. I noticed that as the months went by, I did become stronger, with more energy. I started to run again and have joined the Sistership Dragon Boat team, which is made up entirely of breast cancer survivors. I still have lingering side effects from my treatment that occasionally get in the way of my fitness routine, but I have learned to be much gentler with myself. I know that tomorrow is a new day and that I have the opportunity to adjust my activities. I now consider exercise as a prescription—another important aspect of my treatment.

I would encourage women who are going through breast cancer treatment and recovery to be physically active. Seek out opportunities to be active. Ask a friend or family member to support and join you. When someone expresses their interest to help you—skip the offer of lasagne as you probably have a freezer full of casseroles anyway—let them know that what you really could use is a walking buddy or someone to drive you to yoga. I promise you that you will feel better for it!

Walking—It's That Simple

Walking is one of the safest and easiest physical activities you can do. It doesn't need to cost anything because you don't need to purchase a pricey gym membership or expensive gym equipment. And you can walk almost anywhere at anytime, no matter the season.

Walking is good for everyone. Walking has been shown to help prevent some types of cancers and to reduce the risk of cancer returning as well as reducing the risk of stroke, diabetes, heart disease and osteoporosis. It can lower your blood pressure and reduce harmful cholesterol. Walking can even increase your flexibility. Regular walking will help you maintain a healthy weight, especially when combined with nutritious meals. Walking is the simplest way to improve your overall health, and most people can do it.

Research suggests that walking may be especially important for women with breast cancer or women who have had breast cancer. One study[25] found that women who walked less than 90 minutes per week experienced more symptoms of fatigue by the end of their cancer treatments. In the group classified as "high walkers," no women reported fatigue. However, 17 percent of women in the "low walkers" group reported severe fatigue at the end of the program.

Walking to stay physically active during your breast cancer treatments may reduce your fatigue and nausea. It may also improve your quality of life and overall health. Unfortunately, most women with breast cancer are not active enough to see

---

25 Mock, V., et al. (2005). "Exercise manages fatigue during breast cancer treatment: A randomized controlled trial." *Psycho-Oncology*, 14, 464–77.

these benefits, either because they are experiencing side effects from treatments, don't have enough time in their day or because they are struggling to get motivated to be active.

Walk This Way!

Most people walk as a form of physical activity. In our studies, we have found that walking is the activity that survivors prefer most to do.[26, 27] Survivors of other cancers such as non-Hodgkin's lymphoma, ovarian cancer and endometrial cancer also prefer walking as their main way to be active. Of course, if you jog or lift weights, these activities are also beneficial to your health. But if you are new to physical activity or are admittedly out of shape, walking is one of the best exercises to start off with. Start slow, and walk at a pace that is comfortable for you.

The following are some reasons that survivors may prefer walking over other types of physical activity.

✔ You can walk anywhere and at any time.

✔ You can walk at a moderate intensity that is practical and realistic.

✔ You don't need a personal trainer.

✔ You can walk according to your own schedule.

✔ You can alone or with other people.

Everybody is walking. Use a step pedometer to get a step ahead!

---

26 Vallance, J., et al. (2013). "Rural and small town breast cancer survivors' preferences for physical activity." *Int J Behav Med*. Epub ahead of print.

27 Vallance, J., and Courneya, K.S. (2012). "Social cognitive approaches to understanding exercise motivation and behavior in cancer survivors." In G. Roberts and D. Treasure (Eds.), *Motivation in Sport and Exercise:* Volume 3 (299–326). Champaign, IL: Human Kinetics.

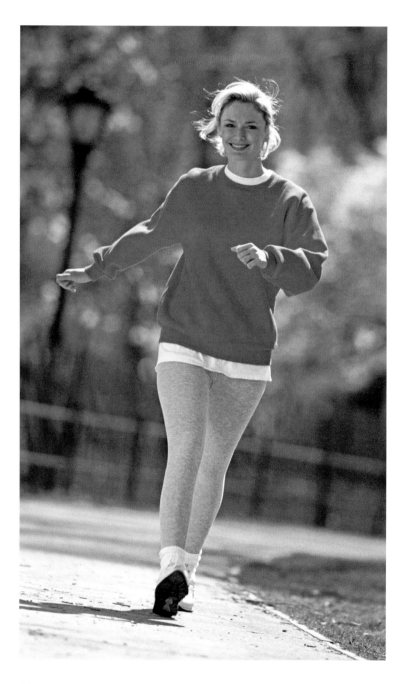

Do I Have to Walk?

Absolutely not. The types of physical activity you can do are endless. The key is to find an activity that you love to do. Skiing, hiking, swimming, golfing…it all counts.

The Culos-Reed Health and Wellness Laboratory at the University of Calgary recently developed an evidence-based yoga program for cancer survivors.[28] The program is known as Yoga Thrive. Scientific research studies of this seven-week yoga program found that yoga participants improved their quality of life and emotional well-being (improved mood and decreased stress) compared to survivors not doing the yoga program. Yoga participants also reported improvements in some of the side effects associated with cancer treatment.

What Is Brisk Walking?

It is important that you walk at a brisk pace, or at a moderate intensity. Have you ever walked to the point where you found it slightly more difficult to maintain a conversation with your partner, you started to sweat a little bit and you could feel your heart beating faster? Or perhaps you have had to walk quickly to the bus stop so as not to miss the bus? That's walking at a brisk pace.

There really is a difference in the effects of normal or light walking (e.g., strolling around the house, walking to the water cooler at work) compared to brisk walking, or walking like you were late for an appointment. And there is some good research evidence for picking up the pace in your steps.

---

28 Culos-Reed, S.N., et al. (2006). "A pilot study of yoga for breast cancer survivors: Physical and psychological benefits." *Psycho-Oncology*, 15, 891–97.

One research study[29] conducted at the University of Alberta gave people a pedometer and a stopwatch. Participants in the study were taught to increase their stepping rate (or pace) by 10 percent. For example, if a participant took 2000 walking steps in 30 minutes, that person then aimed for 2200 steps in 30 minutes. The researchers found that increasing the walking pace by 10 percent significantly improved cardiovascular fitness levels among the participants. And that's from walking only 10 percent faster. Could you pick up the pace by that much?

If you count your steps using a pedometer, there is a simple way to determine if you are getting the right amount of daily physical activity. Research has found that walking 3000 steps in 30 minutes is about the equivalent of being physically active for 30 minutes at a moderate intensity level.[30] Of course, as an alternative, you can also accumulate 1000 steps in 10 minutes at three separate times throughout the day to achieve the same 3000 steps. Using a watch or a stopwatch on your walk can help you determine if you are walking fast enough. Count how many steps you do in 10 seconds and then multiply that by 6 to determine how many steps you do in one minute. Then you can multiply that number by 30 to see how many steps you are doing in 30 minutes.

What do we mean by "walking faster"? Walk with a purpose, so that your heart rate increases slightly, and you might even sweat a little bit. Your breathing should increase, but you should not be out of breath. Buy yourself a pedometer so you can monitor your steps. Keep in mind that a pedometer can't track how fast you are walking—that is up to you and how you feel.

---

29 Johnson, S., et al. (2006). "Walking faster: Distilling a complex prescription for type 2 diabetes management through pedometry." *Diab Care*, 29, 1654–55.

30 Marshall, S., et al. (2009). "Translating physical activity recommendations into a pedometer-based step goal: 3000 steps in 30 minutes." *Am J Prev Med*, 36, 410–15.

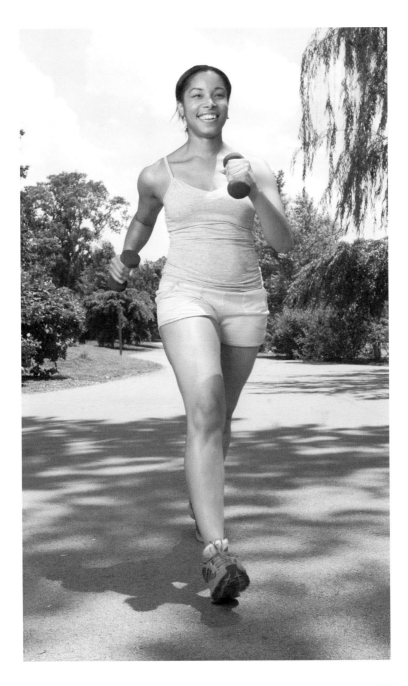

Here are some tips that can help you walk faster.

✔ Look ahead of you instead of at the ground.

✔ Keep your back straight rather than hunched over.

✔ Tighten your abs to help you stand tall.

✔ Relax your shoulders, bend your arms at the elbows and gently swing your arms front to back. But don't swing your arms too high.

✔ Keep your strides the same length. Take faster, not longer, steps.

✔ If you have an iPod, download some songs with a fast beat, head out for your walk and try to walk to the beat.

Of course, you can't always be stepping around and walking like you were late for an appointment. Your schedule might not allow that to happen if you are at work and don't have the proper shoes for walking, or you might be looking after your children all day. Know that your walk does not have to be planned or scheduled around a running track, walking path or trail. Walking can be done in shorter increments. Some days you just have to try to get in as much movement as your time allows.

A lot of research has emerged recently showing that spending too much time sitting is not good for your health. It's not good for your waistline or your mental health, and sitting too much even increases your risk of chronic disease.[31] And so far, we are finding that it may be very important for cancer survivors to limit how much time they spend

---

31 Owen, N. (2012). "Sedentary behavior: Understanding and influencing adults' prolonged sitting time." *Prev Med*, 55, 535–39.

sedentarily.[32] Stand up, take a break and go for a walk. Even if you are walking in shorter increments, you can still walk briskly so that you are getting some moderate intensity activity.

Every step adds up, and every step counts. Here are a few ways you can reduce the time you spend sitting and get some more movement into your day.

- ✔ Take a walk break instead of a coffee break at work.
- ✔ Park farther away from the door of a store or your workplace.
- ✔ Take the stairs instead of the elevator.
- ✔ Use the farthest restroom in the building.
- ✔ Keep moving—pace around or circle the room any time you are waiting for someone or something.
- ✔ Skip the drive-through (e.g., bank, pharmacy). Instead, park your vehicle and walk to the building.
- ✔ Walk over to a co-worker's desk instead of using the phone or email.
- ✔ Walk around the house during TV commercials.
- ✔ Walk to visit your neighbour rather than drive.
- ✔ Play tag with your nieces, nephews, children or grandchildren.
- ✔ Dancing counts, too! Put on some upbeat music and enjoy a twirl.

---

32 Lynch, B. et al. (2013). "Don't take cancer sitting down: A new survivorship research agenda." *Cancer*, Epub ahead of print.

Enjoy Longer Walks

You may have time to add one or more longer walks during the week. These walks may be scheduled or done on the spur of the moment when you have some free time. Here are some ways to fit longer walks into your daily routine.

✔ Form a neighbourhood walking group and walk together in the morning, noon or evening.

✔ Tour the town by foot—check out the flowers, gardens or holiday light displays you encounter along the way.

✔ Explore nature trails in your area.

✔ Register to walk in a charity event such as the Canadian Breast Cancer Foundation Run for the Cure. Plan weekly training walks together.

✔ Walk your kids to school.

✔ Mow your lawn using a push mower.

✔ Walk the golf course instead of using a cart.

✔ Get your walking in while your kids are in activities or sports—climb up and down the stairs at the hockey arena or walk around the ball diamond.

✔ Create an "exercise" playlist on your iPod or iPhone. Put your earphones in and step to the beats.

...add one or more longer walks during the week...scheduled or done on the spur of the moment...

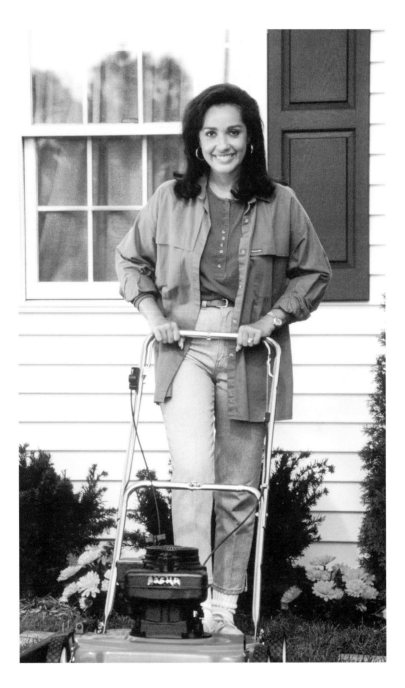

Dr. Laura Rogers

For many breast cancer survivors, regular physical activity may be as important as taking their anti-cancer medication. Multiple research studies have shown that women with a history of breast cancer who engage in regular physical activity can potentially decrease their risk of dying from their breast cancer by almost half. The good news is that physical activity can reduce your health risk while also helping you feel better physically and mentally.

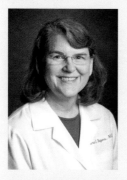 Your oncologist may have advised you to lose weight or prevent weight gain. This is because excess body weight may increase a woman's risk of dying from her breast cancer. Physical activity is important for any weight management program. Importantly, physical activity can help reduce your abdominal fat, which is the fat most likely to increase your cancer risk.

Regular physical activity is now considered by oncology professionals to be an important part of the post-diagnosis survivorship plan. To help you become and remain physically active, start at a level that is safe and gradually increase the amount you are doing. Talk with your health care provider if you have health conditions or cancer treatment side effects that may affect your physical activity program. Find a certified personal trainer with experience working with cancer survivors (especially if you have lymphedema). Check out the internet because the number of online resources is growing every day. For general information, consider expert sites such as the American Cancer Society, American Institute of Cancer Research, and American College of Sports Medicine.

Find friends and/or family to exercise with you and encourage you to stick to your exercise program. Choose physical activities that you enjoy. Integrate more physical activity into your daily life. Use a pedometer or another individual monitoring device for motivation and to track your progress. Try out different approaches until you find one that works for you. The improvement in your health and well-being will be worth it.

–Dr. Laura Rogers is a professor in the Department of Nutrition Sciences and internal medicine physician in the University of Alabama Weight Loss Medicine Clinic. She has published several ground breaking studies that explore the role of physical activity in breast cancer survivors.

"...women...who engage in regular physical activity can potentially decrease their risk of dying from their breast cancer by almost half.

Making It Happen

Research has shown that setting goals will help you start and maintain your physical activity program. Setting goals will also help you monitor how much physical activity you are doing. Write down your goals (use the tear-out pages we have provided) and put them on the refrigerator or another place that you will see daily so that your family can view the goals and help you achieve them.

Use the following "SMART" guidelines when setting goals.

- ✔ **Specific:** Determine exactly what you are going to do and how.
- ✔ **Measurable:** Measure your progress.
- ✔ **Attainable:** Set a goal that is within your reach, not an impossible dream.
- ✔ **Relevant:** Set a goal that is relevant and rewarding.
- ✔ **Time frame:** Set a reasonable time frame that allows enough time to reach your goal.

Remember to reward yourself when you have reached a goal. Treat yourself with something that you enjoy, such as taking a long hot bath, buying that book you have been wanting to read or buying a new pair of runners.

Continue to Set Goals

Continue to set weekly goals until you meet the recommended goal of being physically active at a moderate level for at least 30 minutes a day for at least five days a week. If you are physically active at a vigorous level, aim to do this at least three days a week.

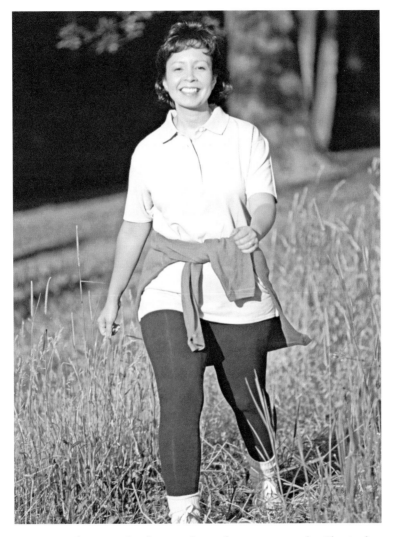

You can keep track of your physical activities in the Physical Activity Calendar that we have provided at the end of this book. Record the physical activities you are doing and the time you spend doing each activity. Use pages 66 and 67 to list your physical activity goals.

ACTIVITY 5: SET A GOAL

STEP 1

Write a goal for the week by filling in the blanks.

Starting on _____ (day of the week),

I'm going to _____ for _____ minutes.

I'm going to do this _____ days this week.

STEP 2

Write down what else you need to do to meet this goal. For example, you may need to buy some walking shoes or invite a friend to start walking with you. Maybe you need to buy an exercise video or borrow one from your local library, or call your local fitness centre and sign up for a class.

_____

_____

_____

_____

_____

_____

STEP 3

Write down how you will reward yourself if you meet your goal this week.

_____

_____

_____

_____

_____

_____

_____

EXAMPLE OF A WALKING GOAL

Starting on Monday, I'm going to walk for 30 minutes. I'm going to do this five days this week (Monday to Friday).

I'm going to phone my friend Kari to see if she will walk with me after work or at lunch time.

If I follow this schedule for two weeks, I will buy myself a new pair of walking shoes.

Use these two pages to write out your physical activity goals.

_____

_____

_____

_____

_____

_____

_____

_____

_____

_____

_____

_____

_____

_____

_____

_____

_____

_____

_____

_____

_____

_____

_____

_____

_____

_____

_____

_____

_____

_____

_____

_____

_____

There may be times when you don't feel able to exercise. The goal is to be as active as you comfortably can be. Try exercising when you have the most energy. Even a few minutes of gentle stretching can help you feel better.

–Canadian Cancer Society

Where the Rubber Hits the Road!

The next part of this book talks about strategies for living a healthy lifestyle that includes physical activity. We all have reasons for not fitting daily physical activity into our busy schedules. To top that off, side effects from your chemotherapy treatments may prevent you from wanting to be active. Keeping up a regular physical activity routine can be difficult. However, there is an easier way to accumulate your physical activity.

Physical activity experts propose the 10-minute solution. You don't have to set aside an entire half-hour to do your physical activity. On those especially busy days, try building in 10 minutes of physical activity three times a day. For example, you can do some simple activities for 10 minutes in the morning, take a 10-minute walk during lunch and walk around the block for 10 minutes in the evening. And there you have your 30 minutes of physical activity. It's that simple!

Be Barrier Aware

Sometimes we think that physical activity has to be something that is structured, rigid and time consuming. Our challenge to you is to think outside the box and start thinking about physical activity differently. You don't have to go to the gym, run on a treadmill or sign up for an aerobics class to achieve a healthy level of physical fitness. It is critical to build physical activity into your everyday routine.

Here are some simple changes that may help you get the physical activity minutes you need (I bet you didn't think some of these choices were physical activities!).

- ✔ Instead of getting coffee from the coffee machine at work, walk to the nearest coffee shop and get a coffee on your coffee break.

- ✔ Purchase a pedometer, clip it on and monitor your steps. Knowing how many steps you take during the day is a great motivator to take more and more steps.

- ✔ Purchase a Wii Fit or similar video game system for your family. Rather than sitting on the couch, you can get up and moving.

- ✔ Combine physical activity with another activity you enjoy, such as walking on a treadmill while watching TV or reading.

- ✔ Take a 10-minute walk after meals. Ask family members or a friend to join you.

- ✔ Set your clock alarm to go off every hour; walk for two minutes each time it goes off.

- ✔ Use physical activity as transportation. That is, ride a bike, walk to the bus stop or walk to work.

- ✔ Wake up 30 minutes earlier in the morning and get some physical activity in. Then go to bed 30 minutes earlier.

- ✔ Schedule physical activity into your daily routine rather than waiting to see where physical activity will fit in.

Dr. Katia Tonkin

There is a lot of emerging data that physical activity is very beneficial to patients going through treatment for breast cancer. Even
during chemotherapy, physical activity can help with tiredness
and mood, and from studies done here at my cancer centre, it has
been shown to improve survival. The activity does not have to

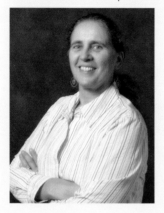

be anything out of the ordinary, and
walking is sometimes the easiest
and best activity, but doing weights
as well as cardio is beneficial. I recommend patients stay active during and
after their treatment, and along with
a healthy diet, this is the best advice
that we can give to improve well-
being and outlook for our patients.
It is simple to do and makes an enor-
mous difference for our patients.

–Dr. Katia Tonkin is a professor and medical oncologist at the
Cross Cancer Institute in Edmonton, Alberta. She specializes
in breast and gynecological cancers. She is a member of the
Northern Alberta Breast Cancer Team

Even during chemotherapy,
physical activity can help with
tiredness and mood, and...it has
been shown to improve survival.

ACTIVITY 6: OVERCOMING BARRIERS

Our daily routines are full of tasks that prevent us from being physically active. Make a list of the barriers in your daily life that keep you from being physically active. Then think about some strategies you can use to overcome these barriers. Discovering the barriers is the first step in overcoming them.

Example of a barrier: *My kids always need my attention after work, so I never have time to do any physical activity.*

Strategy to overcome the barrier: *Ask my partner or a friend to look after the kids for 30 minutes on weeknights while I go for a walk with the girls.*

BARRIERS

Barrier 1:_____

Barrier 2:_____

Barrier 3:_____

Barrier 4:_____

STRATEGIES

Strategy 1: _____

Strategy 2: _____

Strategy 3: _____

Strategy 4: _____

Treatment Day

On the day that you are scheduled for treatment, you may want to avoid strenuous physical activity. However, you may find that going outside for a short stroll can be refreshing. The side effects of chemo treatment tend to hang around for a few days. So on these days, it might be a good time to rest. It all depends on what you can tolerate. You are in charge, so listen to your body, and take a break if your body is telling you to do that.

Better yet, use these days to do some easier activities such as light walking or gentle yoga or Pilates. Try doing some stretching exercises. Becoming more flexible will only help you in your physical activity choices. It may also help prevent you from feeling sore or stiff from the tasks you need to do.

Here are some light activities that you can do on the day of your treatment and on the days when you might not be feeling so well immediately after your treatment day.

- ✔ Watch your favourite movie and do some stretching in front of the TV.
- ✔ Buy or borrow a yoga DVD and try some of the yoga poses.
- ✔ If you have a dog, take it for a walk.

You may find that even these light activities are too difficult to do. If you feel that way, remember, sometimes being active may not be what your body needs at that time. You may need to just curl up in bed and read a good book. You can always try to be more physically active when you feel up to it.

During and Between Cancer Treatments

The common side effects, such as nausea and vomiting, of chemotherapy or other treatments can prevent you from being active. The side effects depend on the type of chemotherapy you have been prescribed. There is some evidence that physical activity can help reduce some of these side effects, but the evidence is inconclusive.

However, chemotherapy side effects don't have to stand in the way of being physically active. The best strategy is to plan around the times you feel the side effects the most.

❏ Are there certain times during the day that your side effects seem to limit you?

❏ Are there other times of the day you tend to feel better?

You can try to be active when the side effects are not present. For example, if you feel nauseous in the morning and fatigued in the evening, try doing your physical activity in the afternoon. Another strategy is to start off your physical activity very slowly. Once you get moving and are active, you may find that the side effects you are experiencing go away.

There is some evidence that physical activity can help reduce some of these side effects...

Cold Weather

We're not strangers to cold weather! But you can still do your daily physical activity. If the weather is too cold for your liking, find an indoor activity that you enjoy. You can join or start a mall-walking club or visit your local fitness centre.

Here are some cold-weather survival tips.

- ✔ Ease into it. Start off your walk slowly to give your muscles a chance to warm up.

- ✔ Walk at a moderate or slow pace. Winter roads and paths can be icy. The longer your walking stride, the higher risk you have of falling. Match your walking stride to the path you are walking on.

- ✔ Bring water. Dry winter air is dehydrating, and we do sweat in the wintertime, so be sure to drink water.

- ✔ Stay safe. In bad road conditions, walk where there is little or no traffic. Go to parks, shopping malls, bike paths, high school tracks or streets that draw few vehicles.

- ✔ Wear three layers of clothing. It's better to overdress. You can always remove a layer of clothing if you get too hot.

- ✔ Avoid cotton. Wear clothes made out of material that will keep moisture away from your skin, such as wool.

- ✔ Wear gloves. Wearing gloves, a hat and a scarf will help you keep warm. If your hands, ears or head get really cold, go inside.

- ✔ Wear outdoor footwear. Lightweight hiking boots are a good option. But avoid wearing heavy hiking boots that are meant for mountaineering.

- ✔ Don't layer your socks. Wearing more than one pair of socks can form blisters on your feet. Use thin wool socks designed to keep your feet warm.

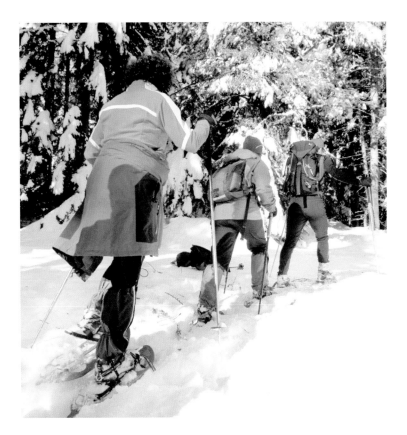

There is no such thing as weather that is too cold—there's only the failure to dress properly!

If the weather is too cold for your liking, find an indoor activity that you enjoy.

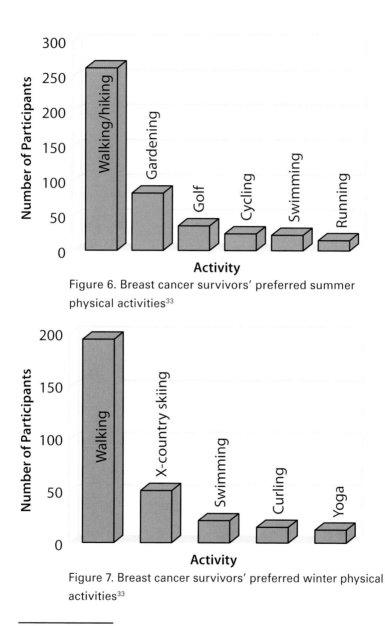

Figure 6. Breast cancer survivors' preferred summer physical activities[33]

Figure 7. Breast cancer survivors' preferred winter physical activities[33]

33 Vallance, J.K., Lavallee, C., Culos-Reed, S., & Trudeau, M. (2013). Rural and small town breast cancer survivors' preferences for physical activity. *International Journal of Behavioral Medicine*, 20, 522–528

ACTIVITY 7

Write down some places where you can be physically active when it is too cold outside for you to walk.

1. _____
2. _____
3. _____
4. _____
5. _____
6. _____

Fatigue

Feeling tired is one of the main reasons women give for avoiding physical activity when receiving breast cancer treatment. A large percentage of women who have had breast cancer report that they experience fatigue. It seems counterintuitive, but physical activity is a powerful strategy to beat feelings of fatigue. Many women believe they should relax or take it easy when they are feeling fatigued, but the scientific research tells us an opposite story.

When you are feeling tired, that is the time to get outside or get up and be active. Being tired, or fatigued, can get you into a vicious cycle. When you feel tired, you usually want to rest and lie down. But studies show that doing this only makes you feel more tired. The strategy is to break the cycle with a healthy dose of physical activity.

In research studies with breast cancer survivors, walking and other forms of physical activity have been found to reduce tiredness. Studies suggest that as little as 30 minutes of brisk walking per day reduces symptoms of tiredness. Remember, the 30 minutes can be broken into three, 10-minute sessions per day—you don't have to do the 30 minutes at one time.

If you are tired, here are a few tips to maintain your physical activity.

✔ Notice the days and times of the day when you feel fatigued. Then be active at a time when you feel the least tired. Experts suggest that being active in the morning is a good strategy to avoid having fatigue disrupt your schedule.

✔ Ease up on your activity and do what you can tolerate. If you are doing any moderate or vigorous intensity activity, and you are feeling tired after a few days, decrease the level of intensity or decrease the amount of time you workout.

✔ It is important to get your body moving. If you don't feel you can handle a higher level of physical activity, visit your local YMCA or a community fitness centre and jump into the pool for a light swim. The cool water will be refreshing, and you will be moving around.

...be active at a time when you feel the least tired.

Other Health Issues

As we talked about earlier, women diagnosed with breast cancer are now being encouraged to be physically active even while undergoing chemotherapy treatment.

Besides facilitating your recovery from breast cancer, physical activity is recommended in the management (and prevention) of many health conditions not related to your cancer diagnosis. The benefits of living a physically active lifestyle are tremendous!

Physical activity can help you with the following physical or psychosocial issues you may be dealing with:

- ✔ arthritis
- ✔ fibromyalgia
- ✔ heart disease
- ✔ diabetes
- ✔ high blood pressure
- ✔ menopausal symptoms
- ✔ osteoporosis (brittle bones)
- ✔ overweight/obesity
- ✔ psychosocial health
- ✔ self-esteem and confidence.

If you have any other medical or health problems, you should ask your doctor or oncologist before starting any type of physical activity program. If you are given the go-ahead, start being active at a level that you can tolerate and that is enjoyable to you. If you have pain or aches in a particular area on your body, avoid doing the physical activities that cause you discomfort.

Lisa A. Workman, M.A., B.P.E., CSEP-Certified Exercise Physiologist

During my career, I have had the opportunity to work with many breast cancer patients and survivors. Cancer treatment is an exhaustive process, when patients are encouraged to be inactive, so it is not surprising that most people think of exercise as a positive way to regain vitality and strength only *after* treatment. But exercise can also be a valuable form of self-care *during* treatment, both enhancing quality of life and improving clinical outcomes. I would highly recommend that all breast cancer patients and survivors participate in as much physical activity as they are able to do, not only for their physical health but also for their mental well-being.

The research is pretty clear that physical activity helps before, even during, and after treatment; so I encourage people to begin a progressive exercise program as soon as they feel able, working on slowly increasing both the frequency and duration of their sessions. Even just 10 minutes or more of cardiovascular exercise most days of the week will make a big difference. As a society, the idea that survivors should be "resting" after treatment is so ingrained that I find people just need to ease back into physical activity. Walking is one of the easiest forms to incorporate after treatment—you don't need to hit the gym or do anything too exotic, just moving helps. As you become stronger, that is when I encourage people to consider supplementing with resistance exercises.

Cancer survivors may find working with a qualified exercise professional will help with their exercise program design but, perhaps even more importantly, can also help them keep motivated. Motivation to keep moving must be linked to overall outcomes, and that should be continually reinforced in people's minds, so working on goal setting helps ensure success.

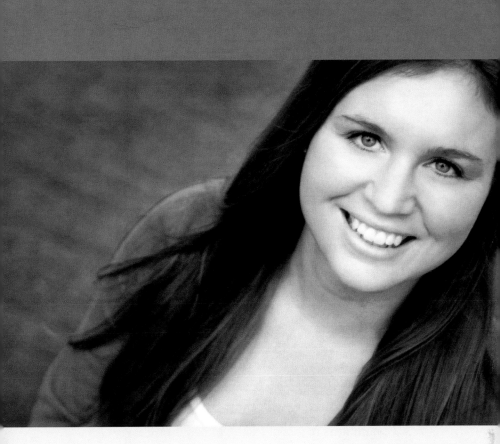

"Even just 10 minutes or more of cardiovascular exercise most days of the week will make a big difference....[you] just need to ease back into physical activity.

Listen to Your Body

If you notice any of the following symptoms while you're doing a physical activity, stop and call your doctor:

- ❏ an irregular pulse (heart seems to skip a beat)
- ❏ shortness of breath or difficulty breathing
- ❏ extreme fatigue
- ❏ unusual muscle weakness
- ❏ joint or bone pain (besides the everyday aches and pains some of us have)
- ❏ leg pain or muscle cramps
- ❏ chest pain
- ❏ sudden onset of nausea (feel like you are going to vomit), dizziness, blurred vision, fainting
- ❏ fever or shaking with chills
- ❏ numbness or loss of feeling in hands or feet

Stretching properly and drinking plenty of fluids can prevent many of these symptoms. It is important to drink fluids before, during and after physical activity so you don't get dehydrated. Try to drink one extra cup of water for every 30 minutes of moderate physical activity. You may need more fluids when it is warm and humid outside. Take a water bottle with you and keep sipping!

Try to drink one extra cup of water for every 30 minutes of moderate physical activity.

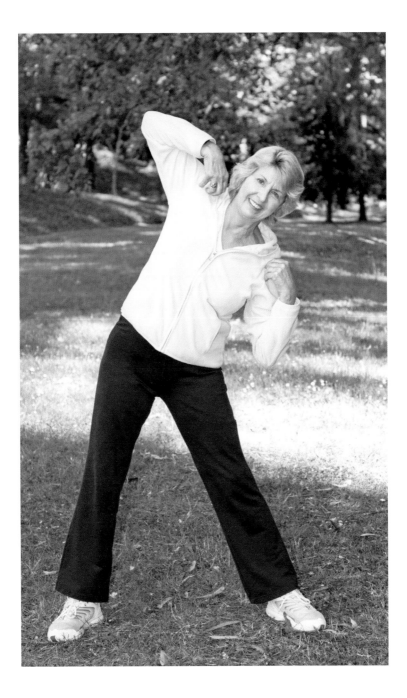

Final Thoughts

We hope you have found this book useful. For the past 15 years, we have been working with cancer survivors and finding ways to improve their fitness, as well as ways to be physically active. We know that facing a breast cancer diagnosis and treatments is challenging. Through all the survivors we have worked with, we consistently see how powerful physical activity is for changing people's lives. We have seen how physical activity changes the way someone looks, their attitude, and their general outlook on life.

We hope you will find your own ways to be physically active. There isn't one magic trick that works for all. You need to find the activities you enjoy and the passions you want to pursue. We can almost guarantee that if you start engaging in a physical activity you really don't enjoy, your physical activity program will not last very long. Life is too short to stick yourself on a treadmill when you just don't want to be there. Taking the dog for a walk at the park is something that is much more appealing than a treadmill! Our challenge to you is to make regular physical activity a part of you, and a part of your life. You will not regret it.

We welcome your feedback on this book. We also welcome you to share your story with us. How has physical activity helped and changed you? How do you stay physically active? Never hesitate to contact us. You can email Jeff at jeffv@athabascau.ca and follow him on Twitter, @jeffvallance.

Good luck!

Appendices

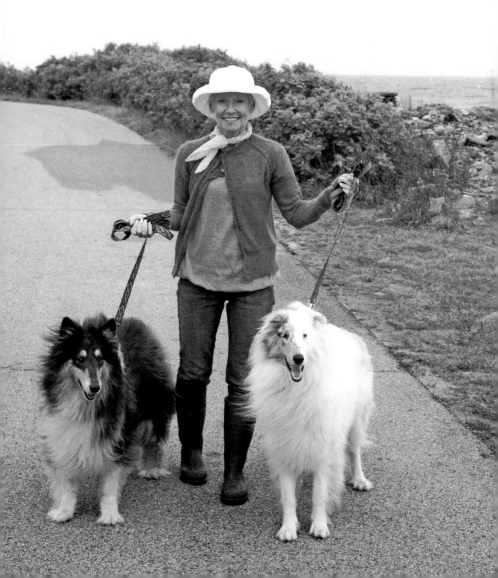

Sample Walking Program

Week		Warm Up	Activity	Cool Down	Total Time
Week 1		During each week, do at least three walking sessions on different days, outlined below:			
sample week	Session 1	Walk for 5 minutes	Then walk fast for 2 minutes	Then walk slowly for 5 minutes	12 minutes
	Session 2	Repeat above pattern			
	Session 3	Repeat above pattern			

Continue with at least three walking sessions during each week using the progression below.

Week 2	Walk for 5 minutes	Then walk fast for 4 minutes	Then walk slowly for 5 minutes	14 minutes
Week 3	Walk for 5 minutes	Then walk fast for 6 minutes	Then walk slowly for 5 minutes	16 minutes
Week 4	Walk for 5 minutes	Then walk fast for 8 minutes	Then walk slowly for 5 minutes	18 minutes
Week 5	Walk for 5 minutes	Then walk fast for 10 minutes	Then walk slowly for 5 minutes	20 minutes
Week 6	Walk for 5 minutes	Then walk fast for 12 minutes	Then walk slowly for 5 minutes	22 minutes
Week 7	Walk for 5 minutes	Then walk fast for 14 minutes	Then walk slowly for 5 minutes	24 minutes
Week 8	Walk for 5 minutes	Then walk fast for 16 minutes	Then walk slowly for 5 minutes	26 minutes

Week	Warm Up	Activity	Cool Down	Total Time
Week 9	Walk for 5 minutes	Then walk fast for 18 minutes	Then walk slowly for 5 minutes	28 minutes
Week 10	Walk for 5 minutes	Then walk fast for 20 minutes	Then walk slowly for 5 minutes	30 minutes
Week 11	Walk for 5 minutes	Then walk fast for 22 minutes	Then walk slowly for 5 minutes	32 minutes
Week 12 & beyond	Walk for 5 minutes	Then walk fast for 24 minutes	Then walk slowly for 5 minutes	34 minutes

Tracking Your Steps

Seeing really is believing! We have provided a Physical Activity Calendar (page 90) to help you monitor your progress. Use the calendar to record the total time you spend on moderate and vigorous intensity physical activity each day. If you have a pedometer, you can also use this calendar to record the steps you take each day. Research has found that people who track and monitor their health behaviours (such as physical activity or diet) are more likely to stick to the behaviour. Follow these instructions to help you:

1. Record the total daily minutes you spent doing moderate physical activity.

Moderate-level physical activity makes you breathe harder but without feeling out of breath. If you are exercising at a moderate level, you should start to sweat after 10 minutes of activity.

For example, if someone saw you walking at a moderate intensity, they would think you were late for an appointment. Other examples of moderate intensity activities include doubles tennis, easy bicycling, Pilates, yoga, easy swimming and folk dancing or any other popular dances such as Zumba or hip hop.

Record the number of minutes you spend doing moderate physical activity in the calendar under "Mod:" For example, if you did yoga on one day (at a moderate intensity) for 15 minutes and walked briskly for 25 minutes during that one day, that is a total of 40 minutes of moderate physical activity. You would record the time as follows:

Day 1

Steps: *8482*

Mod: *40 mins*

Vig:

This is where to record the minutes you spent doing moderate physical activity.

Moderate-level physical activity makes you breathe harder but without feeling out of breath.... if someone saw you walking at a moderate intensity, they would think you were late for an appointment.

2. Record the total number of minutes you spent doing vigorous physical activity in one day.

Vigorous-level physical activity makes you sweat right away, and your heart beats very quickly. You should find it difficult to talk when you are active at a vigorous level. Examples of vigorous intensity activities include taking part in an aerobics class, jogging, swimming laps, hard bicycling, playing soccer or singles tennis.

Record the time, in minutes, that you spend doing vigorous physical activity in the calendar under "Vig." For example, if you jogged on the treadmill for 15 minutes, then you would record it as follows:

Day 1

Steps: *8482*

Mod: *40 mins*

Vig: *15 mins*

This is where to record the minutes you spent doing vigorous physical activity.

You should find it difficult to talk when you are active at a vigorous level.

Physical Activity Calendar

Day 1	Day 2	Day 3
Mod:	Mod:	Mod:
Vig:	Vig:	Vig:
Day 4	Day 5	Day 6
Mod:	Mod:	Mod:
Vig:	Vig:	Vig:
Day 7	Day 8	Day 9
Mod:	Mod:	Mod:
Vig:	Vig:	Vig:

Day 10	Day 11	Day 12
Mod:	Mod:	Mod:
Vig:	Vig:	Vig:
Day 13	Day 14	Day 15
Mod:	Mod:	Mod:
Vig:	Vig:	Vig:
Day 16	Day 17	Day 18
Mod:	Mod:	Mod:
Vig:	Vig:	Vig:
Day 19	Day 20	Day 21
Mod:	Mod:	Mod:
Vig:	Vig:	Vig:

Physical Activity Monitors

Electronic physical activity monitors are becoming very popular; you might even own one. Perhaps you have heard of the Fitbit or the Nike Fuelband. These are just two of the devices that you can purchase to help track and monitor your activities. There are lots to choose from, and all perform a similar function. Most of them count your steps and provide you with an indication of how much physical activity, along with the intensity of activity (mild, moderate or vigorous) that you do each day. Many of these devices sync to your wireless device (such as your iPhone), allowing you to view the different activity intensities and walking steps you have done up to that point in the day. Often your data is presented to you in a graph format so that you can see how you are progressing day by day.

These devices all do a suitable job at tracking your activity, and they are fairly accurate at estimating how much energy you are expending and how much you are moving.[34, 35] But, most importantly, all of these devices give you feedback. They provide you with a benchmark for how active and inactive you are throughout the day. Wearing any one of these devices can provide you instant feedback and motivation to start moving more. Just imagine, if you get 3000 steps one day, you'll want to shoot for 4000 the next.

The pedometer is still one of the cheapest and most effective ways at helping you put one foot in front of the other...more often! These devices can be purchased at your local sporting goods outlet or running/walking store. And given the research

34 Lee, JM., Kim., Y., Welk, GJ. (2014). Validity of consumer-based physical activity monitors. *Med Sci Sports Exerc*, Feb 5, Epub ahead of print.

35 Takacs, J., Pollock, CL., Guenther, JR., Bahar, M., Napier, C., & Hunt, MA. (2013). Validation of the Fitbit One activity monitor device during treadmill walking. *J Sci Med Sport*, Oct 31, Epub ahead of print.

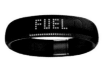 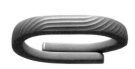

Nike Fuelband   Fitbit   Jawbone Up24

evidence showing the health benefits of walking for breast cancer survivors (such as reduced risk of recurrence, less fatigue), using a pedometer makes sense.

Just like when you are watching your dietary intake with the hopes of losing a few pounds, tracking and self-monitoring are the most important influences on whether you succeed or not. The same goes for physical activity. So track away...

Here is an example of the types of information you can get on your mobile phone from an activity monitor. This example is from the Fitbit, which is one of most common activity monitors available at your local sporting goods store. Other activity monitors produce similar information. Not only can these monitors track your activity time, sedentary time, steps and calories, but you can also create your own social

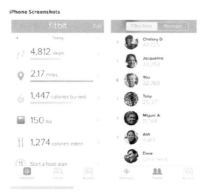 network to see what your friends are doing, which can make for some fun challenges.

Image taken from www.fitbit.com

Further Resources

Alberta Cancer Foundation
www.albertacancer.ca

Alberta Innovates–Health Solutions
www.aihealthsolutions.ca

American Cancer Society
www.cancer.org

Breast Cancer Society of Canada
www.bcsc.ca

Canadian Breast Cancer Foundation
www.cbcf.org

Canadian Breast Cancer Foundation, CIBC Run for the Cure
www.runforthecure.com

Canadian Cancer Society
www.cancer.ca

Canadian Institutes of Health Research
www.cihr-irsc.gc.ca

Nutrition and Physical Activity Guidelines for Cancer Survivors
http://onlinelibrary.wiley.com/doi/10.3322/caac.21142/full

The Ride to Conquer Cancer
www.conquercancer.ca

JEFF VALLANCE, PH.D.

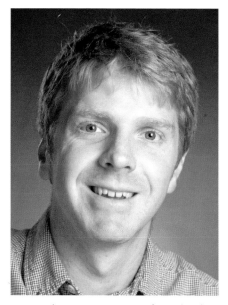

Dr. Jeff Vallance is an Associate Professor in the Faculty of Health Disciplines at Athabasca University in Alberta, Canada. He currently holds a Tier II Canada Research Chair in Health Promotion and Chronic Disease Management as well as a Population Health Investigator Award from Alberta Innovates–Health Solutions. He is an adjunct assistant professor in the Department of Medical Oncology at the University of Calgary. He received his Ph.D (2007) in Physical Education and Recreation from the University of Alberta. Jeff completed his undergraduate degree in the UBC School of Human Kinetics (2000). Jeff's research program explores physical activity, sedentary behaviour, and related psychosocial health outcomes across the cancer context. He is also involved in (and leading) several studies to objectively assess sedentary time and physical activity behaviours of cancer survivors. His research also aims to develop and evaluate strategies to facilitate physical activity among cancer survivors. Jeff lives in Medicine Hat, Alberta, with his wife and three young children.

KERRY COURNEYA, PH.D.

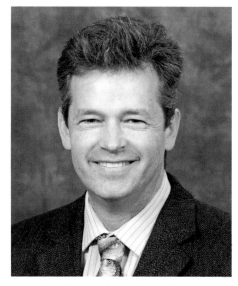

Dr. Kerry Courneya is a professor and Canada Research Chair in the Faculty of Physical Education and Recreation at the University of Alberta in Edmonton, Canada. He received his B.A. (1987) and M.A. (1989) in physical education from the University of Western Ontario (London, Canada) and his Ph.D. (1992) in kinesiology from the University of Illinois. After spending five years as an assistant/associate professor at the University of Calgary, he accepted a position at the University of Alberta in 1997. His research interests include both the outcomes and determinants of physical activity as well as behaviour change interventions. He has co-authored the American Cancer Society's physical activity and nutrition guidelines and the American College of Sports Medicine's exercise guidelines for cancer survivors. He was the guest editor for a special issue on Physical Activity in Cancer Survivors in *Psycho-Oncology* in 2009 and was lead editor for a special volume on Physical Activity and Cancer in the book series *Recent Results in Cancer Research* (2011). Kerry has published over 300 papers on the topic of physical activity and cancer. Kerry lives in Edmonton, Alberta, with his wife. They have two children who are both attending university.